I0830003

ONE CHANGE AWAY

Your Guide to a High
Performance Life

BRANDON HALL

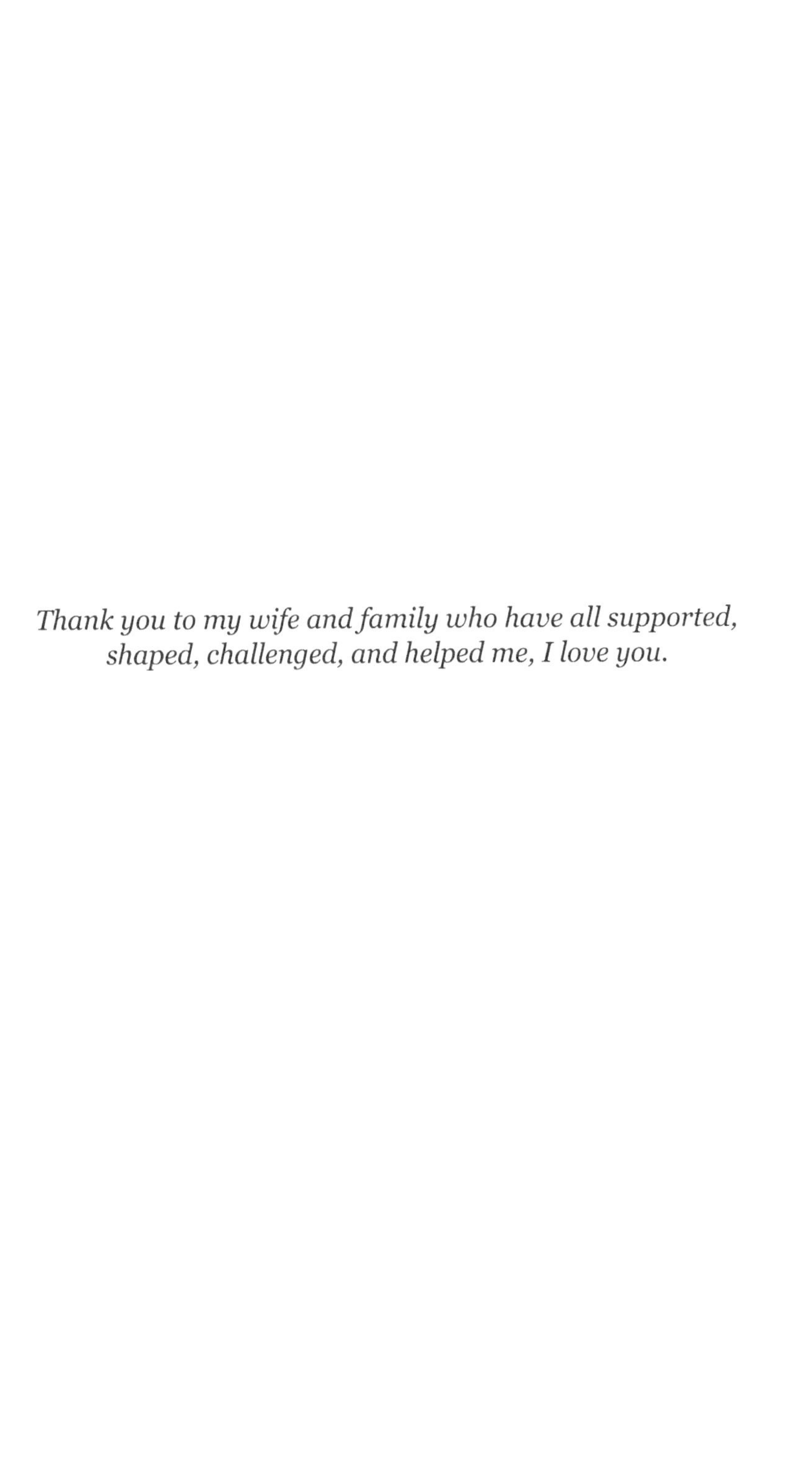

*Thank you to my wife and family who have all supported,
shaped, challenged, and helped me, I love you.*

CONTENTS

PREFACE

Here is the origin story behind *One Change Away*: it all begins with my non-traditional upbringing. My dad and my mom were and continue to be great parents to me. They did everything they could to provide the most for my siblings and I, but, through various events of life, their divorce took place when I was 8 years old. After that, my weekends consisted of traveling to my mom's house for a weekend and back to my dad's for the week to go to school. Changing schools every other year throughout middle school left me with very few established friends, and this took a toll on my social abilities and social confidence. I would tell myself I was not worth other people's time and quickly became a very shy and quiet individual. I ended up living a lifestyle that would follow the trends of most children with divorced parents with low to middle income who live in trailer courts: I did not respect myself and found a connection in "living it up on the weekends". I'd stay out all night with my 'friends', and even though I pretended like the parties and the mischief was what I wanted, I knew deep down that I was lying to myself and creating a front where I could safely hide behind.

Although I was not living a fulfilling lifestyle, I had always been an active person and participated in football all through high school. Given the physicality of the sport and my lack of taking care of my body, football led to a major injury where I dislocated my knee cap. Even though it was extremely painful - I was sobbing when I arrived home that night - I was more concerned with never being able to play the sport I loved so deeply rather than crying from the pain in my leg. This was one small turning point regarding my mindset. As I went to physical therapy, I began to see the results of consistent work, and my knee was getting better. I started to learn something through the commitment and hard work that the therapy forced me to work on: only with dedication can your life begin to change.

It was now my senior year in high school and I had to register for my final semester of gym class. My school didn't offer me a huge variety of classes; I remember looking down at the list and struggling between 'team sports' and 'weightlifting'. Did I want to take team sports, stay in my comfort zone, and play the same games that I had been playing since middle school? Or, did I want to take a risk and try something new, something that I knew challenged me? I decided to try weightlifting out. The first few days of class had passed and it was now time to max out - I had to demonstrate just how much I could lift; I stepped up to the bench press, laid down and, at 6'1 and 155 pounds, I grinded and gave everything I had to push the 95 pounds off my chest. There it was: as an 18-year-old, I benched 95 pounds as my one rep max, and I had to give it my all to even make that happen. As I sit down to write this, it still seems crazy to think about the progress I have made since then.

 After showing up to class every day, following the programs that were provided, and surrounding myself with the people who took the class seriously, I went from that 95-pound bench press to a 185-pound one rep max in a single month. Are you kidding me?!?! For the first time in my life, these dots connected. I found that if I put in consistent work and simply showed up, the results will come naturally. That mindset sticks with me to this day.

In the time I spent in that weight room, I physically, mentally, and spiritually developed. The work ethic that I discovered altered my attitude towards school work (although this realization was a bit too late: I graduated high school with a 2.9 GPA and only received an 18 on my ACT), towards my relationship with God and trusting in Him since He created every moment that led to me finding my passion, and continues to lead me each day. I was made into a new person; the old me could not keep up with the new me; I was so focused and determined that nothing could get in my way. These moments laid the foundation for a year that would create more change than I could imagine.

Success is a word that can have a different meaning to each person; while it is commonly used or seen as a measure of the amount of money one has in their bank account, I see success as the lifestyle one is living. When I wake up, am I pursuing something that I am passionate about? Am I being the caring and loving individual that God made me to be? Am I becoming a better person, being self-aware as to where I need to improve? These are all measures of success for me, and I believe it is possible that if we pursue these types of standards for ourselves, then we can provide far more for the people in our lives than what we thought possible. The money that we all strive for will arrive naturally as long as we are truly passionate about these standards. During this time of change, I dove into several books that laid out this model for a successful life, and I'll note these titles later on in this book. I am not a big reader, so for me to take a book and read it cover to cover says a lot about the value of any book, so I highly recommend getting all of them!

The most progressive and proactive year of my life was the summer after I graduated high school. I worked at a car wash where I vacuumed cars, but my dad was able to help me secure a different job with Fed Tech, a waterjet manufacturing company, by August of that year. With his help, I began a different type of manual labor position that required early mornings and a hard work ethic. Even though I was at the bottom of the ladder in the company, the small business owner made it a point to talk to me and ask me how I was doing every time I saw him. The respect he showed meant a lot, and I saw that the stereotypical "successful person" did not have to be a jerk or big-headed, and that changed the ideology of "nice guys finish last" that I'd believed before. A successful person does not have to be mean or selfish; rather, a successful person consistently shows up, persists through the trials of life, and is ultimately looking towards the betterment of those around them.

During that summer of change, I began to enjoy waking up early and took a sense of pride in it. I began to learn that most successful people are early risers: they are able to complete half their day's work before most people are even awake, eliminating all distractions and therefore creating a more efficient and productive day.

Another lesson that I learned within that productive year was that just showing up eliminates the majority of the feelings of defeat or doubt that I had. It's human nature to overthink every little detail of one's day - to stress about the seemingly-enormous task list to the point that, before we even arrive to work, we are already overwhelmed. What if I told you that it could be simpler? Well, it is! How easy is it to pull out your phone and scroll through social media? Of course, you just take your phone out and do it. We do not think about, oh, now I need to dig in my pocket, pull my phone out, have it scan my finger to unlock or enter a password, click on the app itself, wait for it to load and finally I can scroll through social media. For some reason, our brains don't see all these little steps as stressful tasks. Yet, for something like going to the gym, we break it down into 50 steps that need to take place in order for us to arrive and get a workout in. Instead of this overthinking, just get up and go. Get ready and head out as soon as you arrive, and you will feel like you accomplished something. You already invested that time to show up, and now you are in an environment where others around you are getting after their goal. Then, after the workout, as the endorphins are running through your body, you're feeling good, and you're ready to attack the day.

Here are the final highlights of that year of major progression: I found that same work ethic that I established at the gym also carried into my performance at my job and in my online college courses. I continued to work out so that I could try out for the football team at the University of Wisconsin River Falls (UWRF). After all that hard work, showing up, studying, and training, my days consisted of weightlifting, working, and 2-3-hour coffee shop visits after work to complete my school work. Soon after, I was accepted to UWRF, solidifying my goal to become a first-generation college student. During my time at UWRF, I met my girlfriend and now-wife, Brooke, participated in collegiate football, attended Florida International University in Miami for a semester, and earned two degrees, one in marketing and another in economics within the traditional four-year timeframe. My life of living-it-up-on-the-weekends had completely changed. This is only the beginning, and I hope that my story can show that no matter what you have gone through or what you have done, it is never too late to overcome the odds and change for the better, regardless of your "why". You can make a decision *today* to take the next step in becoming a high-performance individual in every way, from the mind to the body.

This book's purpose is to give you the tools to create a driven, high-performance life: financially, spiritually, physically, and emotionally. It is a part of the Starting Fresh Development Plan -

you can learn more at startingfreshdevelopment.com. Coupled with the advice, testimony, and plans laid out in this short book, you're going to be well-equipped to achieve all of your goals.

I did my best to explain this in a way that was as concise as possible, only leaving applicable information that can be implemented in your life, starting today! I look forward to what is to come, and I thank you from the bottom of my heart for investing your time towards reading this book.

Chapter 1

GOALS

We need something to strive toward, it starts here.

Without establishing goals, life can be unfocused. It seems to become a reactive game of insanity, and while each day has the potential to be a good one, the purpose of the day will most likely fade, bringing you down and draining your energy. While there are many ways to establish goals and review them, some people may create too many goals, which can be overwhelming. On the other hand, others might not even know where to start. Both are okay! Below are some tips to help create a foundation of realistic, simple, and effective goals:

- Before writing goals, write a few affirmations about yourself to set a positive tone. Always use "I am" when writing/saying these affirmations
  - Example: I am an optimist; I look for the good in EVERY situation
- Ask yourself this question: What key areas in life are important to you and/or could use improvement?
  - Some examples could be:

- Family
  - I am closer with my family, reaching out to them on a consistent basis to reestablish lost relationships
- Spirituality
  - I am growing with God each day, loving just as He loved me, and doing the best I can to fulfill His purpose for me
- Health
  - I am the healthiest individual I know, always learning how to take better care of my body, always showing up to the gym, whether I feel like it or not
- Public Speaking
  - I am attending a Toastmasters meeting where I speak clearly, with confidence. I want to use emotion as I speak to gain the attention of those who hear me so that they listen to me
- Business Ideas
  - I am the owner of an ecommerce business that provides great products to my clients, my clients to trust that we have the best prices and great quality

- Happiness

- I am a happy individual that knows that I am in control of my emotions; it is up to me to decide how I handle situations that arise within my life, no one can take this away from me

Writing positive affirmations and visualizing what you want for yourself is an effective goal-making skill. In order to become who you want to be, you have to *know* what you want to be. Write down as many things as you can!

Now that you have an idea as to what makes an effective goal, before reading any further, jot down the keywords that come into your mind when you think about who you want to be in six months to a year. In that time, you could dramatically change as a person! Having a clear idea about who you want to be and defining what is important to you is a fundamental part in becoming a successful individual, no matter what your definition of success is.

With a general outline as to who you want to be, we can now move on to thinking about the next steps: what would you like to spend your time doing?

We have one life to live and I believe your ultimate meaning in this world is far greater than most believe to be possible. So, what's stopping you from becoming the best version of yourself? What are some things that are holding you back? The most common factors are time and money. Let's spend some time discussing each of these two factors to unpack how each can be detrimental to growth.

Time

Time is the most valuable thing in our lives, and while many of us work the 9-5's, it's important to note how is your time spent outside of the workplace. This can be a touchy subject - sometimes looking yourself in the eye and realizing that you're not making the most of your time can be emotional and challenging - but it important to evaluate it because the same 24 hours are used by every other person you look up to. And, if they can achieve what they have with their time, so can you - believe that to the deepest depths of your heart.

Everyone's heard of a budget - it's a system where you track how you spend money. Have you ever considered tracking how you spend your time, a resource that's even easier than money to waste? What blows my mind is the fact that the average American watches 5 hours of television each day (Hinckley 2014). If we can work towards limiting that wasted time and utilizing a little bit of it towards being engaged in our passion, I believe a shift would occur where the positive energy within us could not be contained. Social media is another consumer of our time, and although it can be used to run a business or create a following, the mindless scrolling is where the danger lies. There has been plenty of times where I go on my phone and start scrolling and soon a whole half hour has passed, and I have not gained or improved in any way. Like financial budgeting, there is always room for entertainment and activities, and the same can be said for television or social media. However, the key is to keep it in balance and have your time management align with your purpose and goals that you've now worked on establishing.

Money

Another factor that most people find holding them back is money. Financial management was never a skill that I excelled at, but through resources like Dave Ramsey's Financial Peace University and books like *Unshakeable* by Tony Robbins and *Rich Dad Poor Dad* by Robert Kiyosaki, and Dave Ramsey's *Complete Guide to Money*, I've found strategies that work for me. But I also have to give a lot of this credit to my wife, she has very strong determination and dedication when it comes to the world of budgeting and being money-conscious. Maybe you are already responsible with your money, or you are that support that someone needs in regards to finances, that is great! Keep learning and developing, become even more of an expert. If you do not have a foundation or that supporting individual, that is okay! It is a skill that can be attained; for starters, I highly recommend you purchase Dave Ramsey's *Complete Guide to Money*. Use the knowledge that is provided in his book and pair it up with the app that he and his team put together called *EveryDollar*, you will be off to a great start!

While it might feel overwhelming to learn how to handle money, educating yourself has never been easier. It used to be that, if we wanted to learn or become skilled in a subject or service, we could not get this information without going to school and earning a formal education. But through the evolution of YouTube and Google, you can type in what you want to know and educate yourself on anything: Facebook marketing tips, how to create a successful Instagram post, or how to write a book. A whole world of information is lying within the phones we look at every day and the computers we use, and the best part is that a lot of it is free. Through the use of the internet, starting a business does not require a physical location 100% of the time anymore, if finances are a stopping point in regards to you pursuing your goals an online business is a great way to make it happen with a relatively small amount of overhead costs.

After breaking down and hopefully eliminating some stress about time management and finances, ask yourself this: What is it that I am most interested in? What would I wake up and start working on even if I was not paid? My friend Joe asked me this a few years ago, and ever since then, I've used these questions to help guide my actions and maintain a certain standard of living an excellent life. My hope is that you will pursue the same because you are full of greatness. We can all achieve so much more than we think is possible if we start to redefine what we "should" be doing, what the "norm" is, or what "reality" has to be like. There are far too many great ideas that are being suppressed by the doubters who do not believe in the greater power within themselves. Do not listen to the doubt in your mind that tells you there is not enough time or money, and do not let others bring down the ideas and creativity that are flowing within you.

Chapter 2

MINDSET

The power to create a winning mindset is within you.

Your mind is very powerful. It has the ability to do amazing things; just look at people like Kyle Maynard, Wim Hof, and David Goggins. These individuals overcame tremendous odds using their minds; Kyle climbed Mount Kilimanjaro without any legs or arms, Wim ran a marathon in shorts and sandals above the Arctic Circle, and David completed 4,030 pull ups in 17 hours. While these feats are amazing and hard to even comprehend, one thing is clear: the mind is the variable that allowed them to succeed. If you can get ahead of the negativity that your mind naturally creates, then you're on the right track to creating a winning mindset. You have the confidence to tell yourself that, no matter what you're trying next, you are the best man or woman for the job. Although the situation at hand might not turn out exactly the way that you imagined it would, have faith that you can handle anything that comes your way. This amount of confidence is not easy - it's not created in the blink of an eye, but cultivating it will lead you towards a winning mindset.

A winning mindset can only be truly attained when you lean in to a positive, healthy community - they will support you and are essential to your success. In this next section, we'll take some time to dive into the topic of relationships: the nourishing ones and the poisonous ones.

Before we continue, take a moment to revisit the items you wrote down, think about the affirmations you have for yourself, and once again ask yourself this question: who do you want to become? Understanding this answer will help you start to make decisions about the types of people you should surround yourself with. Sometimes, it's easy to devalue how much the people you spend time with impact your life. You might think to yourself, "even though my best friend is constantly negative, it's ok because I am a positive person. They won't change that about me!" What you might not realize is that your friends and family shape who you are, so spending time with people who are consistently positive, outgoing, goal oriented, loving, polite, humble, and confident will help to ensure that you are also these things. Whoever you decide to spend most of your time with you become, you will believe what they believe, and you will be on the same track to follow where they are going. To create a strong, resilient winning mindset, find a community that supports where you want to go, *your* goals, *your* mindset, and *your* habits. My hope for you is that you can find a community that will push you toward the person you would like to become. A few resources that I have used in the past include Bible study groups, Toastmasters, and apps like Eventbrite, MeetUp, Shapr, and Instagram. Even though it can seem intimidating to join new communities, most of the people you meet are excited to help you.

There have been times where I felt like I did not have much to offer. But when I leaned in to my communities, I quickly learned that friendships and relationships, when given time, even out. Even if you feel like you're asking for help without giving anything in return, give it time. You will absolutely have the chance to pay it forward - eventually, one of your friends will be in a pinch, and you'll have the opportunity to support them the way that they supported you. People in search of winning mindsets are all on the same team: when you start seeking them, you will be happily surprised how many people you will find.

Another factor that determines your mindset is the content you consume. Have you ever noticed how 90% of the headlines that you see are negative? This is a purposeful choice. Companies understand that drama sells, and the idea that something is going horribly wrong in someone else's life might make a consumer feel better about himself. Consuming so much negativity can stop a winning mindset from fully developing.

It only takes one person with the right mindset to reach out and help create positive change. Think about the factors that lead to a winning mindset. Many of them are out of your control, but there are just as many that you *can* control: what media you consume, who you spend time with, and what you spend your time doing. The message is this: you can control certain incoming factors and paying close attention to them is so important. Pay attention to the music you listen to. I love music - I listen to it constantly, and I enjoy a everything from rap to classical, but the type of music I listen to does not consist of drugs and misogyny; it consists of overcoming odds, becoming a better person, and knowing there is a God that surrounds me through the best circumstances and the worst circumstances, and who loves me far more than I can ever imagine. To sum up, pay attention to what you're filling your life with.

Something that has also helped me succeed is to listen to at least one podcast every day. There are podcasts about literally everything: from faith, to marketing, to history, to nutrition. There are podcasts out there for everyone. I like them because I learn such valuable information, and most of the time, they're completely free. Obviously there is YouTube, but SoundCloud is another app that offers thousands of podcasts. Think of them as a free class without homework, and sometimes the people who are speaking on podcasts are some of the best in their industry.

Let's say that you choose to listen to a podcast every day on your morning commute, and we'll assume that your commute is 20 minutes. This equates to a little over 6.5 hours per week of personal growth and development, and that's not including any additional reading or networking that you do. Big changes are coming your way if you take this approach!

> **Tip**: James Altucher, while speaking with Lewis Howes on the "School of Greatness" podcast made a great point: anytime he learns something new or reads something new, he writes down 10 takeaways from the content. This practice helps with retention and applying the knowledge into your life. Keep a notebook or a notebook app close by and you can easily do this as well!

The main takeaway from this chapter about mindset is this: the individuals who succeeded beyond their wildest dreams spend time cultivating their winning mindsets. They did this by being thoughtful about who they spent their time with, what content they consumed, and they actively spent time learning new things. It is my belief that no single person is better than the next - if someone else has done something amazing, so can you! Your picture of success might not identically match your role models, and you might even be surprised by how your success takes shape, but no matter what, know that you have the power within you to capitalize on the success by using the power of your mind.

Chapter 3

HABITS

Showing up breeds results

Throughout this book we've worked on discovering your goals and the realizing the power of a mind that is truly focused. While fully embracing these two elements is a great starting point, what good are they if they are only utilized once a month? To find success in any form, it takes consistency in showing up, even when you do not feel like. If you are having a hard time visualizing where you want to be, imagine that you are living the life you want, doing what you love, being able to spend time with the people that you want, and having the financial freedom to support your family and the community. Visualizing this with all your strength makes it seem so real that your heart begins to beat harder and faster because it is all possible; believe that to the deepest depths of your heart. Personally, I use these visualizations when I need to motivate myself to get out of my warm, comfortable bed in the morning and go to the gym to train. When I hear my alarm go off, I immediately turn it off, tell myself I am too tired, that I can go tomorrow, and that it will be okay. To overcome this moment, I need to picture myself being stronger, pushing my limits, and fulfilling my goal of going to the gym or participating in some sort of physical activity 7 days per week. Feeling, seeing, and living in those moments before they happen sends energy through me that pushes me into the zone where I cannot be stopped. I've learned that the only thing standing between me and my goal is myself. Through visiting that deep, concentrated vision, I move out of my own way and shut the negative voice in my mind off. Like many things in life, the aspect of personal development is accessed through applying a vision (goals), which then shuts the mind off (mindset), leaving the end result of a habit. As time goes on and your habits feel more natural, you'll notice that you have more energy to achieve your goals. This is especially true as you begin to see real results, whether it be getting a raise, reaching a new one rep max in weightlifting, succeeding during your first networking event, or asking the guy or girl that you have always been attracted to if they want to go out sometime.

Wouldn't it be great to have some guidance in how to reach these goals and create these habits? I've read so many books about this, and in this chapter, I'll distill the most valuable lessons that I've learned, used, and seen work. And, if you have habits of your own that help you to relax, be more productive, get your day started off on the right foot, or help you end your day on a positive note, share them with me on Facebook, Twitter, or Instagram! The more we can provide this information to others, the greater the footprint we can all have in helping others live a meaningful life. Now, let's dive into some great habits!

Let's start by talking about the beginning of each day. Every morning, your first action has the potential to set the tone for your entire day, and this is why either me or my wife begin each day by making the bed. I know there have been a book or two written and even a viral video about this habit, and they all mention the accomplishment that comes with knowing that, if not one thing goes right in your day, at least you can see that bed and know your day started out with accomplishment. I also believe that this creates a focus on doing the little things right; you're making a conscious decision to do something that is not going to be seen by the world, and you will not be applauded for doing it, but in your mind, you know that you completed something. It seems small but beginning each day with an accomplishment is so powerful.

Next, let's discuss food and diet. I firmly believe in healthy living, and the second habit I recommend that will have lasting results is eating quality, nutrient-dense foods. This is rabbit hole for me - I love discussing food and nutrition -, but I will keep it concise and will provide more information in the next chapter.

Have you ever eaten a meal and felt less than your best afterwards? You can make decisions to avoid this feeling. To better regulate the bloated, upset stomach feeling, limit the intake of certain fats, proteins, and carbs. Depending on where they come from, certain fats are quite healthy. To get healthy fats, try eating nuts like pecans, walnuts, and almonds, cook with extra virgin olive oil and coconut oil (sparingly) for smoothies. You can also enjoy coffee and popcorn... yes, popcorn! We all need a fun snack every once in a while, as long as it's not dripping in butter and salt! The nutrient that fuels the body is protein, and it helps with building and repairing the tissues in the body. It's commonly found in high quantities in meat and animal byproducts, such as beef, chicken, and eggs. You can also find a ton of proteins in vegetables like spinach, broccoli, and brussel sprouts, if you are a vegetarian, vegan, or just prefer to limit your meat intake.

There are two key things that people can do to avoid unhealthy inflammation of the body and feeling bad after eating in general: minimizing dairy and eating the right kinds of carbs. Diary, despite the popular myth that claims the richness of calcium and the necessity for proper growth, is unnecessary in the majority of adult bodies. The healthiest type of carbs are complex; they slowly break down within the body, providing sustained energy rather than being deposited directly into our fat stores. Some common examples of complex carbs are sweet potatoes, brown rice, and oats. The other type of carb that many people unwittingly choose to enjoy are simple carbs like white rice, white bread, and flour-based tortillas. These foods and other popular items like soda are tasty, but they trick the body into feeling full and nourished, will in reality, cause an insulin spike in the blood. This spike will eventually come crashing down, leaving the consumer feeling tired, hungry, and craving more of the same food or drink.

Paired with a solid nutrition base, being physically active is the next habit that I've dedicated myself to. Showing up to an early morning workout sets the tone for the entire day: you'll feel more energized, more motivated to accomplish your goals, and physically, your body will be more prepared to properly digest the food you eat.

I know that it can sound impossible to make these changes in your life. Believe me, I know exactly how you feel. I wasn't always confident in my body or actively pursuing a healthy life. But, I have now lived this lifestyle, and the secret to seeing the results you want is persistence and consistency both in the kitchen and in the gym. When I saw the results of putting in work day after day, it all clicked, and from that moment forward, I truly believe if you put in the work, the results will follow. Everyone has one life to live - there are no second chances. For me, these changes saved my life. I believe that anyone, regardless of where you're from, who you are, or what you've done in your life previously, can accomplish their goals if they're willing to put in the hard work.

The third key habit to implement for a high-performance lifestyle is continuous learning and self-education. For example, I consistently read the Bible. As a Christian, I have seen the works that God has done within my life, whether it be my siblings overcoming their drug addictions, my dad being saved and turning his life around after being an alcoholic for many years, my grandparents and their inspiring health and the incredible ways they supported me throughout my life, or the opportunities God has created for me providing me an able body and mind. All of this inspiration enables me to wake up each day knowing He dragged me through the trenches so that I can say today I know where I should be. Because of God's Grace, I am heading toward something that only He can make happen. With this faith, I can continue to work hard even when I feel defeated because I truly believe in God's plan for me.

In addition to the bible, I also read books about business, finances, and self-development. The knowledge these types of books contain is invaluable - and even better, they're affordable! Most books can be purchased Amazon, so to make this easy for you I put together a list top 10 books which is available at startingfresdevelopment.com, all 10 books can be purchased for less than $200 in total. While I'm a firm believer in budgeting, trust me that this investment is worth it. Still not sure if you want to? To put this into a better perspective, I can confidently say that this investment of around $200 taught me more about creating *tangible* results than my college education did.

To conclude this chapter, I want to share my favorite habit. The most effective habit that works and brings great energy to my day is something that I heard from Elliott Hulse. He suggests writing down positive affirmations on notecards and then confidently affirming these things to yourself. I do this during my morning commute, when I can jam out and be a little obnoxious without disturbing anyone. Here's what you should do: take a few note cards and write a few words on each one that represent who you are and what you want to be. For example, one of mine says "Great Communicator!" written on it. Since I have a hard time speaking with emotion and tone behind my words, I overemphasize what I am saying as I speak out loud. As I drive, I tell myself over and over that I am indeed a great communicator, and I put as much emotion as I can into each one. This leaves me feeling confident, energized, and passionate. Leave the cards in the center console or your glove box, and that way, when you drive somewhere, you can remind yourself of your qualities them and generate contagious energy. The key takeaway for this habit is to speak these affirmations out-loud with *emotion*. If you do this one thing consistently, you will notice a difference in your outlook on life, yourself, and even the way people treat you.

BRINGING IT HOME

Whatever your aspirations, they require the trifecta of goals, mindset, and habits coming together to make your dreams a reality. To bring this into perspective, let's take a look at possible outcomes if all three principals are not followed:

Scenario 1: Goals without habits or mindset

Let's say your goal is to read for 30 minutes every day. But, you don't have the correct mindset about your goal, and the habits to make this happen haven't yet been established. On day one, right before bedtime, you dedicate yourself to this goal and successfully read for 30 minutes before lights out. But in the morning, you're tired because you stayed up later, and getting out the door and off to work is a frantic rush. Right off the bat, your day feels off. Perhaps on the way to work, the traffic is stop-and-go and you're fuming in your car, blaming your lateness on the driver in front of you, furious that someone could be so irresponsible. Of course, your lateness is your own fault - had you planned out your morning better, made space in your schedule for your goal, and then enacted what needs to be done to make reading *and* getting your day started, then you wouldn't be so frustrated right now. By the end of the day, you're most likely tired from overcoming the stress in the morning, and your goal of reading for 30 minutes has been placed on the back burner. Had you written the goal down, shared it with others, reviewed it, and planned your day around making it happen, you'd probably be sitting down with a book in your hand right now.

Scenario 2: Mindset without goals or habits

Now, let's flip the script. Let's imagine that you have a great mindset, but that you did not establish goals to meet or habits to follow. We'll stick with the reading example.

When you talk to your friends and family about your reading goals, you're energized and excited. You tell them - and yourself - about all the great books that you're going to read, how much knowledge you're going to gain, and how eager to get started you are. Your mindset is positive - you're feeling great and you believe in yourself.

However, you fail to articulate your *exact* goal. Instead of saying "I will read for 30 minutes each night before I go to bed", you just tell yourself "I'll read more". This vague goal isn't helpful. How will you know if you met it? Maybe your definition of "more" means three hours one day and then three minutes the next. Even if your mindset is positive, creating a goal is so important.

And, so is creating habits that help you attain goals. After you've pinned down what you want to do, habit creation will get you there. If you don't know just what you're trying to accomplish, it's hard to make daily changes to turn that goal into reality. If you say you'll read more, then maybe one day, you carve out an hour after dinner to read. That's great for a day, but how long can you maintain this? Most likely, after a few days, your mindset will start to sour because you won't be seeing or feeling positive results. All that energy that you started out with will being to fade. This is avoidable if you articulate a goal and then set and follow habits that help you achieve it.

Scenario 3: Habits without goals or mindsets:

This scenario is probably most unlikely, but it's still possible. Imagine that you have habits established, but that you don't have a single goal or a goal-oriented-mindset. Most likely, you do have established habits in your day, and you just haven't realized that these habits are more positive than you think.

Perhaps you read the paper, a blog, or a magazine every morning as you drink your coffee or eat breakfast. Or maybe, you listen to a podcast or an audiobook during your daily commute to work. You could create a goal around this habit. You already have a structure in place, and a goal and mindset might organically emerge from this. Instead of just taking these reading habits for granted, you could tell yourself, I want to keep reading every morning, but add five extra minutes of reading every day. At the end of the week, that's 35 extra minutes, and at the end of the month, I'll have read for 150 more minutes.

Why is this beneficial? Why would you do this? If you already have established habits, creating goals around them pushes you to the next level with only a little bit of effort. The action of challenging yourself to be better, to do more, and to do it every day might seem small, but it will extend into other areas of your life.

Imagine that you did this with every habit. Instead of talking to your kids for 30 minutes after school, you talked to them for 35 and put your phone down during that time. Instead of calling your dad every Thursday, you called him every Thursday *and* every Sunday. Instead of training for an hour, you trained for an hour and fifteen, and you challenged yourself with different workouts.

Until you identify a habit and create a goal and mindset around it, your habits might stay invisible. You might miss out on the positive structures that you've already placed in your day. Think about your typical day. Where are the moments that you could do more, or do it better? Take a second to identify something that you do every day, and then try to create a goal and mindset around it.

Depending on your style of communication, this chapter may have been uplifting for some or conflicting for others - it's challenging to admit to yourself where your weaknesses are. I also used to struggle with this, but once I realized that I can achieve so much more when I embrace where my weaknesses are, I now seek weaknesses out. Once I find them, I can conquer them. There may have been moments in the chapter that were more blunt or direct - please don't feel offended or see this as a personal attack. Remember that we are on the same team, and I am here for you! I am here to help you reach your goals, and sometimes that takes speaking truthfully. It's important to surround yourself with individuals who simultaneously support you and keep it real and honest. I am here to personally support you, and I want you to check out startingfreshdevelopment.com to get signed up and we can connect one-on-one over the phone, via email, skype, or even in person! Through our meetings, I can provide the best resources for you and be there to support and provide insight regarding your personal, professional, and spiritual questions.

Chapter 4

NUTRITION

Make your effort to show up worth it

We've spent time discussing habit creation, which is a great transition into our next topic: nutrition. When talking nutrition, many people immediately assume that the conversation is heading in one direction: dieting. I refuse to use the word 'diet'. Rather than limiting ourselves, we are taking out the bad and adding the good. Understanding nutrition is a process that leads to eating healthier, not restriction your body from nutrients that it might need. Taking the following steps and applying them into your life will have a positive impact on how you feel. We're not just creating a mentally healthy mindset, but also working to create a physically healthy body. Some of the athletes that I have known from playing college football would eat just about anything to put up weight - I want to talk more about the dangers of this later, and hopefully inspire both athletes and non-athletes to consider healthier food choices. I want you to feel like you can get up and go without feeling bloated, heavy, or slow at any time. All of that starts here, with nutrition.

I uncovered this vital information years after I began working out. The information in this chapter (and throughout this entire book) has been gathered throughout the past 6 years, and I am giving you the straightforward and simple way to go about nutrition. These steps happen before going to the gym and putting up the weight. This approach takes consistency and persistence, but the results will be well worth it!

In chapter 3 of *One Change Away* we talked a little about this. We focused on creating habits, and this new information can help you start to create healthy habits as soon as the next time that you go to the grocery store.

Let's start with the basics: the three main macros are fats, proteins, and carbs. We'll focus first on fats. There are many different kinds of fats that you can consume: these are saturated fats, trans fats, monounsaturated fats, and polyunsaturated fats. The ones to avoid are saturated and trans fats. The fats that are healthy to consume are monounsaturated fats and polyunsaturated fats. These fats are found within the following foods:

- Nuts (Almonds, Walnuts, etc.)
- Avocados
- Flax Seeds - blend with your protein shakes
- Fish

- Chia Seeds - great source of fiber
- Extra Virgin Olive Oil

Unsaturated fats are good for your heart, skin, nails, and hair. They contain omega 3, 6, and 9, which our bodies cannot produce on its own, but are essential for health. Therefore, 3, 6, and 9 must be added into our diets. Sometimes, these can be difficult to add in, especially if, like me, you're not preparing fish every day. That's what omegas are often supplemented because it is so difficult to reach the recommended daily amount. Imagine that you're in the store, contemplating what kind of omega oil to buy. Here's some knowledge that might make your decision easier: Focus on consuming DHA (docosahexaenoic acid), which supports brain function (by over 90 percent relative to other omega-3s!). Fish oil supplements usually have less DHA relative to EPA (eicosapentaenoic acid) and APA (alpha-linolenic acid), so when it comes to looking for your own supplement options, I would highly recommend finding one with a DHA focus. We receive enough APA through proper nutrition on a daily basis (if you apply the information within this chapter) because it is plant based - eat your vegetables are you're covered! EPA, a marine based omega-3 fat just as DHA is, provides greater support than APA but still has far less of an impact than DHA.

Fat is often seen as a bad thing, and too much of it, especially if it is saturated or trans-fat, can be. But, it does not have to be if you consume the right foods. Earlier in this chapter, I noted that some individuals, whether they are athletes or not, will consume anything to put on weight to become stronger. While it is true that you cannot become stronger without putting on weight, there are two types of fats that our body produces depending upon what we consume and how much of it we consume: external and internal. The most common type of fat our body holds is subcutaneous. This is the fat that we see in weight loss commercials - it is right underneath the skin, and so we call it "external" fat. The second type of fat is visceral, and this is the fat that can be thought of as "internal" because it surrounds our organs. Visceral, internal, fat is far more dangerous than external because it can go undetected and then affects body function. Someone who looks great, maybe even has a six pack, can be unhealthy because of the visceral fat that has built up due to poor food choices. That's what choosing healthy fats is so essential in being a healthy person. With the most complicated macro nutrient covered, let's move onto the topic of protein.

Protein is essential: it creates the building blocks of our bodies. and without an adequate amount of protein, your body will not perform at its peak potential. These building blocks are built with amino acids, and, put simply, they create muscle growth (protein synthesis), promote fat loss, and help the body recover from physical activity. There are 9 essential amino acids which your body cannot make on its own, so they must be consumed with proper eating habits:

- histidine
- isoleucine
- leucine
- lysine
- methionine
- phenylalanine
- threonine
- tryptophan
- valine

The recommended daily amounts will depend on your age, gender, and weight. I track my amino acid consumption and recommend that you do as well! The calculator that I use is at www.globalrph.com, the other 11 (or 12) amino acids are considered non-essential because they can be made by your body. As you can see, protein is clearly important. Understanding which foods contain which amino acids will help you have the healthiest body possible. Take a look at the following list for examples:

- Eggs (provides all nine essential amino acids)
- Beef (supplies iron to the body and provides all nine essential amino acids)
- Chicken (a great lean protein option)
- Beans (filled with fiber and most contain all essential amino acids)
- Fish (contains Omega oils)

If you're on a tight budget and your food choices allows it, I recommend eating eggs. Be prepared to get creative - eating a ton of eggs can get old quickly, but there are so many different ways of cooking them that you can keep it interesting! You can make meals like skillets or hash, omelets, scrambled eggs, or egg bake.

Beans are also inexpensive, and they go a long way. Pair that with some ground beef to make chili in a crockpot and you should have dinner made for the week after just a few minutes of prepping! My hope is, with an understanding as to why protein is essential for the body, you will take action and start to purchase and eat healthy foods. But, how much should you eat? That is what we will cover next.

The amount of macros (fat, protein, and carbs) you consume will depend on your personal health goal. This is where you will begin to see the importance of having the fundamentals from One Change Away implemented into your life. For protein, you need to have certain things established before you can know how much to eat. Are you looking to gain size, become stronger, or put on weight? Depending on your answer, it is recommended that you eat 1 gram of protein per pound of your bodyweight. If you are looking to lose weight, the recommended daily allowance states that you should double your protein intake. This helps to maintain muscle mass while also decreasing your body's fat stores. No matter what your goals are, if you are reading this, it means you are looking to either make a change or simply learn more about the topic of nutrition. The key takeaway about protein is that a healthy amount and type of protein promotes an able body and promotes proper growth and recovery.

The last of the macros are carbohydrates; your body breaks these down and turns them into energy. The most important thing about carbs is that there are two kinds: simple and complex carbs. Simple carbs can come from natural sources like fruits and milk, and they can also come from processed foods, like high fructose corn syrup. Processed simple carbs should be avoided, so there are several things that you should scratch from your shopping list! Some examples would include pop, granulated sugar, many of the sauces and condiments we add to our food for extra flavor, and sports drinks. next time you go shopping take a look at the ingredient list, many of the most common items contain high fructose corn syrup.

Because of the way that certain complex carbs are processed, it is best to avoid products like white rice, noodles, and white bread. Did you know that white rice is actually brown rice that has been stripped of all the nutrients? Brown rice is definitely a healthier option. Noodles and pasta are often created with white enriched flour, which is the same product we use to make our desserts - cakes, muffins, baked goods - so the foundation of a typical entree like chicken alfredo or spaghetti is that from an unhealthy dessert. There are great alternatives to noodles out there: quinoa and brown rice, for example, are both grains that taste great! White bread and bread in general should be avoided; there are so many alternatives out there. To understand more about the types of carbs that you're choosing to eat and avoid, you can use the glycemic index, a scale that rates the quality of the carb. The lower the GI number, the better, more wholesome, the option is. To apply this, let's look at a low (55 or less), medium (56-69), and high (70 plus) ranked food according to the GI:

- Low: Raw fruits and veggies
- Medium: Sweet potatoes and whole oats
- High: White bread and white rice

Eating low GI foods and bearing in mind the healthy choices listed about will help you create a new feeling of energy still keeping your body healthy and strong.

When it comes to proper digestion, the body needs fiber, and, per a study conducted at the University of California San Francisco, the average adult's total fiber intake should be 25-30 grams a day from food intake, not supplements. Some of the most common foods that are high in fiber include oats (4g of fiber per cup), lentils (1g of fiber per tbsp), chia seeds (10g of fiber per ounce), almonds (17g of fiber per cup), peas (7g of fiber per cup), and flax seeds (2.8g of fiber per tbsp), the amount of fiber per serving was provided by the USDA. The additional benefit of fibrous foods are that they usually rate low on the GI scale, meaning that your body breaks them down slower, which supplies the body with more energy over a longer time period.

Unsure how to use chia and flax seeds in your diet? One way to consume them are in a protein shake. I use a single serving blender and add frozen fruit, a scoop of protein powder, almond milk, chia seeds, and flax seeds. It makes for a nutrition-packed drink that fuels that body after a workout or day of exercise!

So, now that you have all of this knowledge, you should feel more prepared to stick your fridge and pantry with healthier foods. A really great way to also make sure that you're holding yourself accountable to your nutrient goals is to track your food consumption. MyFitnessPal is a great app that will help you along with this process and can store information that saves you time. If you would like to have me assist in outlining nutrition guidance based upon your goals, please visit startingfreshdevelopment.com or shoot me an email at brandon@startingfreshdevelopment.com and I would love to help you get started on the right foot!

In order to help you avoid the hassle of going through multiple sources for this information, I briefly cover the macro nutrients in this chapter. If you have additional questions or comments let us know at startingfreshdevelopment.com. Others may have the same question, and by bringing the minds of everyone together, we can help to expand everyone's knowledge when it comes to living a successful and healthy life!

Chapter 5

TRAINING

Stronger, Bigger, Faster, Leaner

Alright, here we go! The final chapter for *One Change Away*! Nutrition and training can be labelled as two separate activities, but where they coincide is when you take the goals you created from Part 1 that relate to your health and well-being and apply the knowledge that has been and will be provided in chapters 4 and 5 to create amazing results. Do you want to gain weight? If so, you should be focusing on having a caloric surplus. Lose weight? Then have a (healthy) caloric deficit. Maintain the same weight? Then intake roughly the same amount of calories that you are burning in a day. Your mindset, goals, habit, nutrition and training need to align, and once combined, propel you towards becoming the incredible person that you're striving to be. This chapter specifically focuses on taking *action*. Within the first three chapters, we spent time discussing the importance of being intentional with your goals, shaping the right mindset, and establishing habits that will positively impact your life. These are essential to success but will get you nowhere without a combined action effort. Your life can be seriously impacted if the information is utilized and applied.

Training is all about showing up, regardless of whether it is cold, raining, snowing, or you just do not feel like it. Just get yourself to the gym and make it happen. Now, if you're hurt, then of course, take time to recover - forcing yourself to work out while injured will only hurt you more. However, if you're feeling sore, then make sure to warm-up properly and get your body moving.

Warming Up

There are three simple products that can help you when it comes to warming up properly: a foam roller, a lacrosse ball, and a resistance band. While all three are affordable, I would suggest investing more towards the foam roller. The brand that I recommend is Trigger Point. Their foam roller called GRID is something that I've used almost every day for the last 3 years, and it's still in excellent shape. The reason for this is because it has a plastic base with foam around it, making it sturdier and more durable. Many of the foam rollers out there are only made of foam, and they will start to cave or deform over time. So, spend the extra money up front (around $40), and you will end up saving money in the end and have a roller that really works.

The lacrosse ball is used for breaking up deep muscle tissue. This might hurt a bit, but it's worth it to endure the healthy pain - your muscles will thank you in the end! Some areas that the ball can be used on are your hip flexors, quads, and low back. You want to find the "sweet spot" where you can tell there is extra tightness. Place the ball under the tight area, and then use your body weight and let gravity take its course in breaking up the muscle fascia. Try 30 seconds if you are just starting so that you can get a feel for this. Take deep breaths and relax the muscle. I find that as time passes, my muscle will relax after a few seconds, and then it will relax even more after another few seconds, and that's what we're looking for here: breaking up those tight muscles that have been overworked.

Lastly is the resistance band. This can be used for many things, including a stretch and exercise called the clam shell which warms up the hip flexors. Resistance bands can also be used to loosen up the shoulders and stretch the back. If you're looking for more ways to use a resistance band, instead of trying to explain these through text I believe it would benefit you more to go to YouTube and search *resistance band stretches.* This way, you can get a visual representation of the movements. and have a clearer picture on how to perform the stretches properly.

To finish up the process of properly warming up, try biking for a few minutes with medium intensity, complete a few rounds of dynamic stretching like high knees, power skips, high knee carioca, and butt kicks - this gets your heart rate up, preparing your body for a more intense workout. Warming up is essential. From personal experience, I know that if this is not done consistently, it will lead to injuries and a lack of mobility, which in turn leads to even more injuries. Some bodies may have more limitations or imbalances than others, but that is not an excuse to put warming-up on the back burner. Do yourself a favor and warmup; it only takes roughly 10 minutes.

Movements

Whatever your image is for your strength, your body, and your growth, just know that it is only yours and no one can take it from you. There's no point in comparing your body or your goals to someone else's because everybody is different. Let's say that I want to have Steve Cook's body. Looking at pictures might be something to keep me inspired from time-to-time, but to try to attain his exact appearance will leave me unfulfilled because my body has a separate foundation, is made up of separate genetics, and we ultimately might have different goals. Stop the comparisons! Don't sell yourself short. Instead, figure out your goal and get after it; you CAN do this!

I'm sure by this point, you understand that, if you want to get stronger, you have to be on a caloric surplus. Okay, great, but where's the applicable information to help me reach my goals? Let's take some time to dive into the specifics.

Before getting into the details of the different approaches to training, I want to make sure the applications of the 1 (or 3) rep max (1RM or 3RM) is understood - a 1 rep max is the maximum amount of weight that you can lift for one repetition within a given exercise. This will apply to some compound exercises. Compound exercises are those that require the movement of multiple joints and recruit multiple muscles the "main three" are: squat, bench, and deadlift. Just know that when I'm talking about a 1 or 3RM, it's not the same thing as talking about a bicep curl or a calf raise. Here's a list of common exercises that can be tracked by a percentage of a 1 or 3RM:

- Squat
- Bench
- Deadlift
- Front Squat
- Power Clean
- Snatch
- Barbell Row

- Romanian Deadlift (more common for 3RM)
- Barbell Military Press

Tracking the max weight you can lift will provide a solid starting point for where your strength is. Now, what if you don't even know where to start? For lifts such as the squat or bench press, start with just the barbell, these are typically 45 pounds and are the most functional piece of equipment within any gym. Get a feel for this weight, focus on breathing through each repetition, stay in touch with your body, and then slowly begin to add weight to the bar. You are not there to impress anyone, so don't feel pressured to pile on the weight right away! You are there to work towards a goal and the journey has to start somewhere!

After reading the information within this chapter, you will be able to find your starting point. Instead of blindly going in and putting on a weight that "feels good", you can have a mathematically-backed approach to help you achieve long-term success. For those of you that are just starting out, these last two topics that we'll discuss are proper form and concentric/eccentric movements. Understanding these will bring you greater results as you work towards your fitness goals.

Maintaining proper form varies for each exercise, but there are some basic trends that apply to the three main lifts. Keep the following ques in mind in order to keep your body safe while lifting.

- **Deadlift**: With a neutral spine, chin tucked in, and shoulders back, take a deep breath in. Keeping your core tight, begin to lift the bar off the ground while maintaining a neutral spine on the way up. As you get just above your knees, exhale, bend at the hip, and stand up straight (without locking your knees) as if you were trying to show off your chest.

- **Squat**: Same approach as the deadlift (neutral spine, chin tucked in, shoulders back, core tight) but with the barbell on your back and your feet cemented to the ground. Take a deep breath in and begin sitting back on your heels till your butt drops just below your knees. Keeping the same form, exhale and explode up, but do not lock your knees.

- **Bench Press**: Lay down on the bench with a barbell in your hand. Make sure the back of your head, shoulders blades, and butt are all touching the bench and that your feet are on the ground. Extend your arms. Inhale and begin lowering the barbell. Keep your elbows in and bend at the elbows until the bar touches you, just below your sternum. Then, push the bar up and exhale driving your feet into the ground (yes, you can utilize your lower body to help with your bench press!).

Concentric motion describes when a muscle is shortening, and eccentric motions describes when a muscle is lengthening. The concentric is the "positive" of a lift. If we take the bench press, for example, the concentric portion of the lift happens when you are pushing the bar off your chest. When you push up, your muscles are contracting or shortening. To describe an eccentric motion, imagine a barbell squat. After you've un-racked the weight and begun dropping down into the movement, your quadriceps lengthen. This is an eccentric motion of the muscle and can be considered the "negative" of a lift.

As each of the three main methods for training are explained, keep these terms in mind and know that a positive or negative movement can be prolonged to increase time under tension, which means that your central nervous system will not know what hit it. This helps us 'trick' the muscle memory that leads to plateaus by switching both the exercises you are doing on a consistent basis and the tempo at which you are prolonging the positive or negative motions.

Types of Training

Depending on your goal, there are several different ways to train in the gym. There are three main types of training: power/strength, hypertrophy, and endurance. If your goal is to become stronger, then focus on strength or power training. Are you looking to increase muscle mass and "get big"? If so, then hypertrophy training would be your best bet. If you are looking slim down and improve cardiovascular health, then endurance training should be your primary focus. The good news is that these are not cut-and-dry; these can be interchanged and brought together to make your workouts fit your goals, these training styles will be covered in greater detail later in the chapter.

Strength training will typically consist of 3-5 sets of 1-6 reps at 75% to 100% of your one rep max (1RM) with a 2-3-minute rest period. For example, if my 1RM for a squat is 275 lbs and it's a 4*3 (4 sets of 3 reps), then I will want to lift around 80% of my 1RM at 220 lbs. If you are going to train up to six reps per set, then it would be best to work at a lower percentage of your 1RM at 75%, and vice-versa for the lower 1-3 rep range. The goal here is to make sure the weight is being moved properly and still challenging your limits.

There is a key balance within weight training: that balance is making sure that you're pushing yourself while not being, what some might call, an "Ego Lifter". An Ego Lifter is someone who is showing off, and these are typically the people with the most injuries and imbalances. I have to be honest with you: I've been the Ego Lifter, and I have injured myself. Speaking from experience, do not lift more than your body can handle without proper form.

Remember to listen to your body, be honest with yourself, and do not worry about what others will think; after all, you are on your own journey, just as they are.

Let's move on to talk about hypertrophy. Hypertrophy is the increase of muscle mass or muscle building, and it is probably the most common style of training among men. This is the typical 3*10, but there is some variance within this approach. Although 3 sets are typical, a workout can range from 3-6 sets and 8-12 reps from 50-75% of your 1RM. The most commonly used phrase within this type of training is when someone says they're looking for the "pump" and "mind-muscle connection". The pump is an increase in the blood flow to a targeted muscle group. The mind-muscle connection is the squeezing of the muscle at the top of the motion, like when you flex your biceps at the top of a curl. You may have seen some people look at their muscles while working out; sometimes it is a matter of people checking themselves out, but it also aids in making a connection when you physically see the muscle contracting as you move the weight. Rest periods for hypertrophy-based training should be about 1 minute, which is significantly less than the strength training rest period. This is because of the lighter weight that is used relative to a strength training approach. The lighter weight does not stress your body out as much, but that's not to say you won't be a little sore the next day!

Endurance training is the third common weight lifting method. This type of training focuses on higher reps and supports cardiovascular health. The sets and reps will vary depending on your goal; I have done everything from 1 set of 100 reps to 2 sets of 20, and 5 sets of 15. Like every other approach, it comes down to your goals, testing your limits, and achieving what you want. Just because the typical range is 12-20 does not mean there are no additional benefits (both mentally and physically) for going above 20 reps per set. If you want a good challenge, test the limits and keep on pushing past what you think is your own breaking point within this approach. I think you will be surprised what comes from getting past your own mind and continuously repping it out. The weight within endurance training should be less than what you can handle due to the higher numbers of reps that you'll be performing. The rest periods should also be shorter at 30 seconds to a minute.

In weightlifting, there is a factor that often goes unseen: the amount of time training takes up in a week. Some say it is as much as the equivalent to a part-time job (I believe it is resume-worthy because it shows dedication!). I understand that not everyone has that much extra time, so I can help you create a plan that works within your life. To get started, please visit startingfreshdevelopment.com and click the "Online Training" page to learn more. My programs will save you the hassle of making your own workout which simplifies the process and will help save your time while taking your physical and mental game to the next level!

The training method you choose to pursue should be based upon the goals that you have set for yourself and is dependent upon whether you want to become stronger, gain muscle mass, or improve your muscular endurance. It is also key to know that, when you choose a type of training for your foundation, the other methods can still be integrated in to your workouts. Make sure you stay consistent - without consistency, the results you are aiming for will not happen if you only go when you feel like it or have extra time. Sometimes, we need to make time, and that is where the first three chapters come into play. Regardless of if you train in the morning or in the evening - with the right foundation, you will make it happen. Please do not waste this opportunity: showing up and working hard separates those who look back and have regrets in life and those who look ahead and live a life worth living.

All the pieces of this book come together and create the foundation for a lifestyle movement. When brought together, it can create change in your mindset and outlook, I know it because I live it every day. In the next section, I share how to gain access to some great additional resources to make sure that your journey does not stop here.

ADDITIONAL RESOURCES

This book was intended to be a quick read because I embraced the harsh reality that although many of the books that I have read created change in my life, the time I spent reading only took time away from me taking action and building my own journey.

There are plenty of other resources and help that I would like to provide, feel free to reach out via email at brandon@startingfreshdevelopment.com, Instagram @bolsonhall, or visit the website startingfreshdevelopment.com.

Whether you are looking to make a change in your life that is personal, professional, and/or spiritual I believe that the information provided can be utilized to create a positive impact in your life. Make the most of the momentum you have going right now, do not let doubt stop you from taking your next steps.

www.ingramcontent.com/pod-product-compliance
Lightning Source LLC
Chambersburg PA
CBHW051228250726
48655CB00006B/2659